HOW TO EAT AND BEAT YOUR DIET COMPLETELY

A COMPREHENSIVE GUIDE TO HEAL YOUR METABOLISM, OPTIMIZE WEIGHT LOSS, AND EXTEND YOUR LIFESPAN

Tran Kahle

TABLE OF CONTENT

CHAPTER 1: METABOLISM BASICS..............17
CHAPTER 2: THE SCIENCE OF EATING.........28
MACRO NUTRIENTS AND MICRO
NUTRIENTS...28
CHAPTER 3: SETTING REALISTIC GOALS....40
ESTABLISHING ATTAINABLE WEIGHT
LOSS AND HEALTH GOALS 40
CHAPTER 4: EATING STRATEGIES 47
MINDFUL EATING......................................47
CHAPTER 5: LIFESTYLE INTEGRATION 54
EXERCISE AND PHYSICAL ACTIVITY....54

INTRODUCTION

The Concept of Eating to Beat Your Diet

In a global saturated with fad diets and quick restore answers, the idea of eating to overcome your diet stands out as a fresh and sustainable technique to weight reduction and fitness. This ebook isn't always approximately restrictive consuming or doing away with your preferred meals. Instead, it is about knowledge the complex courting between what you consume and the way your body methods it. It's about empowering you with the know how to make informed decisions that promote a healthful metabolism, support weight loss, and decorate standard well being.

The primary purpose of this ebook is to offer you with a complete guide to sustainable weight reduction and lengthy term health. We will discover the technological know how at the back of metabolism, the position of hormones, the importance of gut fitness, and the effect of different vitamins in your frame. By understanding those standards, you'll be equipped to create a customized eating plan that works for you, helps your fitness goals, and is enjoyable and sustainable in the long run.

WHY TRADITIONAL DIETS FAIL

Traditional diets often promise rapid results however not often deliver lengthy term achievement. Many people have experienced the cycle of dropping weight only to benefit it lower back, once in a while even greater than before. This cycle isn't handiest frustrating but also unfavourable to our fitness. To understand why traditional diets fail, we want to observe both the mental and physiological affects of weight reduction plan.

From a mental attitude, restrictive diets can lead to emotions of deprivation and frustration. When you deny yourself the meals you love, it is most effective a rely of time earlier than cravings end up overwhelming. This can cause binge consuming and a feel of failure, in addition perpetuating the cycle of weight advantage and loss.

Physiologically, conventional diets frequently sluggish down your metabolism. When you substantially reduce your calorie intake, your body is going into survival mode, holding energy through burning fewer energy. This metabolic version makes it harder to lose weight over time and less difficult to regain it once you come back on your ordinary consuming behavior.

UNDERSTANDING THE RELATIONSHIP BETWEEN FOOD AND METABOLISM

Our our bodies are complex biological systems, and at the heart of this complexity is metabolism—the process via which our our bodies convert food into power. This power is critical for the whole lot we do, from the most simple capabilities like respiration and circulating blood, to the extra strenuous sports like strolling and lifting weights. To recognize the way to consume in a way that helps weight reduction and standard fitness, we must first understand the problematic relationship among food and metabolism.

WHAT IS METABOLISM?

Metabolism refers to all the chemical reactions that arise within our our bodies to keep existence. These reactions may be extensively labeled into sorts:

1. Catabolism: The technique of breaking down food molecules to launch power. During catabolism, carbohydrates, fats, and proteins from the food we devour are broken down into smaller units like

glucose, fatty acids, and amino acids. This breakdown releases electricity that the frame makes use of for numerous features.

2. Anabolism: The manner of constructing and repairing frame tissues and storing power for destiny use. Anabolism makes use of the smaller gadgets produced through catabolism to construct new cellular additives, consisting of proteins and nucleic acids, which can be crucial for growth and restore.

The balance among catabolism and anabolism determines whether or not we save electricity as fat or use it for fast wishes. This stability is prompted with the aid of different factors, inclusive of the types of food we eat, our degree of bodily interest, and our hormonal surroundings.

FACTORS INFLUENCING METABOLIC RATE

Basal Metabolic Rate (BMR): This is the range of calories your frame wishes to hold basic physiological functions while at rest, consisting of breathing, circulate, and cell manufacturing. BMR bills for about 6075% of your overall each day power expenditure.

Physical Activity: This includes all movement, from established exercising to normal sports like on foot and household chores. Physical activity can significantly growth your total day by day strength expenditure.

The aim: Sustainable weight reduction and lengthy term health

The Goal: Sustainable Weight Loss and Long Term Health

Achieving weight reduction is regularly visible as a brief term aim, however authentic fitness and lasting consequences come from a sustainable approach. The closing goal is not just to shed pounds but to decorate ordinary properly being and preserve a healthful weight for life. This chapter will lay the muse for know how why sustainable weight loss and lengthy term health should be your number one cognizance and a way to achieve these desires thru mindful eating and lifestyle selections.

WHY SUSTAINABLE WEIGHT LOSS MATTERS

1. Improved Health Outcomes:

Sustainable weight reduction is intently connected to progressed health outcomes. Rapid weight loss regularly ends in muscle loss, nutritional deficiencies, and metabolic slowdowns, that could negatively effect common fitness. In comparison, gradual and consistent weight loss facilitates keep lean muscular tissues, guarantees good enough nutrient consumption, and helps metabolic health. This method reduces the risk of persistent diseases together with heart sickness, diabetes, and hypertension.

2. Long Term Success:

Quick restore diets and intense calorie regulations are not often sustainable and regularly result in yoyo dieting—a cycle of dropping and regaining weight. This cycle can be detrimental to both bodily and mental health. Sustainable weight loss, carried out through balanced nutrients and wholesome behavior, is much more likely to result in lengthy term fulfillment. It promotes a stable and healthy weight that may be maintained over the years.

3. Enhanced Quality of Life:

Maintaining a healthy weight can substantially enhance the quality of existence. It boosts strength ranges, complements physical health, improves sleep fine, and promotes intellectual properly being.

When you cognizance on sustainable weight reduction, you aren't just running in the direction of a number on the scale; you're making an investment in a more fit, happier future.

THE FOUNDATIONS OF SUSTAINABLE WEIGHT LOSS

1. Balanced Nutrition:

A balanced food plan that consists of a variety of vitamins is crucial for sustainable weight reduction. This way incorporating a combination of proteins, healthy fats, complicated carbohydrates, and fiber into your food. Proteins assist maintain muscle mass, healthful fats aid hormone function, complex carbohydrates provide sustained energy, and fiber promotes digestive health.

2. Regular Physical Activity:

Exercise is a essential thing of sustainable weight reduction. It now not most effective enables burn calories but additionally improves cardiovascular health, builds muscle, and enhances temper. Aim for a mix of cardio physical activities (like on foot, walking, or cycling) and power schooling (which include weight lifting or body weight sporting events) to get the first rate effects.

3. Mindful Eating:

Mindful eating involves taking note of what you consume and the way you sense at the same time as consuming. This practice will let you apprehend hunger and fullness cues, lessen overeating, and increase entertainment of your food. Techniques which include ingesting slowly, savoring every bite, and warding off distractions at some point of food can foster a more fit courting with food.

4. Stress Management:

Chronic pressure can cause weight gain and make it tougher to lose weight. Stress management techniques including meditation, yoga, deep respiratory exercises, and adequate sleep permit you to preserve a healthy weight. Reducing pressure also can improve common well being and excellent of life.

5. Consistency Over Perfection:

Sustainable weight loss is ready making consistent, healthful alternatives in place of striving for perfection. It's vital to be patient with your self and apprehend that development takes time. Small, gradual changes on your eating regimen and lifestyle can upload up to full size results through the years.

WHY TRADITIONAL DIETS FAIL

Traditional diets often promise fast weight loss and short fixes, however lots of them fail to supply lengthy time period results. Understanding why these diets fail will let you avoid commonplace pitfalls and adopt a more sustainable method to weight reduction and health.

1. Restrictive Nature

Deprivation and Cravings:

Traditional diets often contain extreme calorie restrictions or the elimination of entire food groups. This deprivation can cause extreme cravings and feelings of being deprived, making it difficult to stick to the eating regimen in the long time.

Nutritional Deficiencies:

Restrictive diets can result in nutritional deficiencies if they put off meals that offer crucial nutrients and minerals. This can negatively effect ordinary health and properly being.

2. Metabolic Slowdown

Survival Mode:

When you notably lessen your calorie consumption, your frame can input a state of "survival mode." This manner your metabolism slows down to conserve energy, making it more difficult to shed pounds and less difficult to advantage it returned once you resume normal consuming patterns.

Loss of Lean Muscle Mass:

Rapid weight loss can bring about the lack of lean muscle tissue in conjunction with fat. Since muscle mass burns greater energy than fat tissue, losing muscle can similarly lessen your metabolic price.

3. Psychological Impact

Allor Nothing Mindset:

Traditional diets often promote an allor nothing attitude, where any deviation from the plan is visible as a failure. This can lead to feelings of guilt and frustration, which may bring about giving up at the food plan altogether.

Disordered Eating Patterns:

Extreme weight reduction plan can sell dangerous relationships with meals, consisting of disordered ingesting patterns like binge eating, yoyo dieting, and emotional ingesting.

4. Lack of Personalization

One Size FitsAll Approach:

Many traditional diets do not don't forget individual differences in metabolism, activity stages, alternatives, and medical situations. What works for one man or woman may not work for some other, leading to frustration and shortage of success.

THE PSYCHOLOGICAL AND PHYSIOLOGICAL IMPACTS OF DIETING

Dieting is frequently approached with the intention of short weight loss, but the results on each the thoughts and frame can be profound and occasionally unfavorable.

Psychological Impacts

1. Deprivation and Cravings:

Restrictive diets that dispose of entire meals organizations or notably reduce calorie intake can lead to feelings of deprivation. This frequently triggers intense cravings for the forbidden ingredients, making it difficult to adhere to the weight loss plan.

2. Stress and Anxiety:

Constantly monitoring food intake and traumatic approximately weight can increase strain and anxiety degrees. This intellectual stress can make weight reduction plan a burdensome and unsightly enjoy.

3. Guilt and Shame:

When dieters unavoidably slip up or take pleasure in a "forbidden" meals, they frequently revel in feelings of guilt and disgrace. This bad emotional cycle can cause emotional consuming and in addition deviation from the weight loss plan.

four. AllorNothing Mindset:

Many diets sell an allornothing technique, wherein any deviation is seen as a failure. This mindset can be discouraging and can lead people to abandon their efforts entirely after a minor slip up.

5. Social Isolation:

Dieting can impact social interactions, as many social activities revolve round meals. People may additionally keep away from social gatherings to stick to their food regimen, leading to emotions of isolation and lacking out on fun studies.

PHYSIOLOGICAL IMPACTS

1. Metabolic Slowdown:

When calorie consumption is notably decreased, the body responds by slowing down the metabolic price to preserve electricity. This metabolic version makes it tougher to shed pounds and less difficult to regain it once everyday ingesting resumes.

2. Muscle Loss:

Rapid weight loss often outcomes within the loss of lean muscle mass together with fats. Since muscle tissues burns more energy than fat, dropping muscle can in addition decrease metabolic charge and make preserving weight reduction greater tough.

3. Nutritional Deficiencies:

Restrictive diets can lead to deficiencies in crucial nutrients, along with nutrients and minerals, in the event that they put off certain meals companies or aren't nicely balanced. This can negatively effect typical fitness and cause symptoms like fatigue, weakened immunity, and negative pores and skin fitness.

4. Hormonal Imbalances:

Dieting can disrupt the stability of hormones that modify starvation and satiety, which include leptin and ghrelin. This can lead to multiplied starvation, decreased emotions of fullness, and problems in retaining weight loss.

5. Rebound Weight Gain:

The combination of metabolic slowdown, muscle loss, and hormonal imbalances often leads to rebound weight benefit as soon as the weight reduction plan ends. This yoyo impact may be adverse to both bodily and intellectual health, as the cycle of losing and regaining weight maintains.

CHAPTER 1: METABOLISM BASICS

Factors Influencing Metabolic Rate

Metabolic rate refers back to the rate at which your frame burns energy to keep simple physiological features, together with respiration, circulating blood, and regulating frame temperature.

1. Basal Metabolic Rate (BMR)

Definition:

Basal Metabolic Rate (BMR) is the range of energy your body desires to keep simple physiological capabilities at rest. It accounts for approximately 60seventy five% of your overall day by day energy expenditure.

Factors Influencing BMR:

Age: BMR typically decreases with age, often due to a lack of muscle tissue and hormonal modifications.

Gender: Men generally have a higher BMR than girls, as they commonly have a better share of muscle tissues.

Body Composition: Individuals with more muscle tissues have a better BMR, as muscle tissues burns extra energy than fat tissue.

Genetics: Genetic elements can affect your BMR, such as versions in genes associated with metabolism and fat garage.

2. Physical Activity

Definition:

Physical hobby consists of all motion, from dependent exercise to everyday sports like walking and family chores. It extensively contributes on your overall each day power expenditure.

TYPES OF PHYSICAL ACTIVITY:

Aerobic Exercise: Activities like on foot, walking, and cycling increase heart fee and burn energy.

Strength Training: Building muscle via weight lifting or body weight exercises can boom your metabolic price via improving muscle tissues.

Non Exercise Activity Thermogenesis (NEAT): This consists of all of the small, non exercising moves you're making all through the day, such as fidgeting, standing, and shifting.

3. Thermic Effect of Food (TEF)

Definition:

The Thermic Effect of Food (TEF) is the electricity required to digest, absorb, and system vitamins from the food you eat. TEF debts for about 10% of your general daily energy expenditure.

Impact of Different Nutrients:

Proteins: Have the very best TEF, as they require greater electricity to digest and metabolize compared to fat and carbohydrates.

Carbohydrates: Moderate TEF, with complex carbohydrates requiring slightly more power than easy sugars.

Fats: Have the bottom TEF, as they're greater with no trouble absorbed and metabolized.

HOW TO BALANCE YOUR HORMONES THROUGH DIET

Hormonal stability is important for maintaining a wholesome metabolism, regulating appetite, and attaining weight loss dreams. An imbalance in hormones can cause various problems, such as weight gain, fatigue, and mood swings. Fortunately, weight loss program performs a good sized function in helping hormonal stability.

1. Incorporate Healthy Fats

Importance of Healthy Fats:

Healthy fats are vital for hormone manufacturing and regulation. They provide the building blocks for hormones and help with the absorption of fats soluble nutrients.

Sources:

Avocados: Rich in monounsaturated fats and potassium.

Nuts and Seeds: Especially flax seeds, chia seeds, and walnuts.

Olive Oil: A right source of monounsaturated fats.

Fatty Fish: Such as salmon, mackerel, and sardines, that are excessive in omega3 fatty acids.

2. Prioritize Protein Intake

Role of Protein:

Protein supports the production of hormones and enables adjust hunger and urge for food by means of selling the release of satiety hormones like leptin.

Sources:

Lean Meats: Chicken, turkey, and lean cuts of red meat.

Fish: High exceptional resources of protein with delivered advantages from omega3s.

Legumes: Beans, lentils, and chickpeas.

Eggs: A whole protein source with critical amino acids.

3. Consume Fiber Rich Foods

Benefits of Fiber:

Fiber facilitates alter blood sugar tiers and helps healthy digestion, that's crucial for hormone balance. It additionally aids inside the elimination of extra hormones.

Sources:

Vegetables: Especially leafy greens like spinach and kale.

Fruits: Such as apples, berries, and oranges.

Whole Grains: Oats, quinoa, and brown rice.

Legumes: Beans, lentils, and peas.

4. Reduce Sugar and Refined Carbohydrates

Impact on Hormones:

Excess sugar and subtle carbohydrates can cause insulin resistance, which disrupts hormonal stability and contributes to weight gain.

Strategies:

Limit Sugary Foods: Cut back on candies, sugary beverages, and processed snacks.

Choose Complex Carbohydrates: Opt for whole grains and starchy veggies rather than subtle grains and sugary treats.

5. Support Gut Health

Link to Hormones:

A healthy gut micro biome is crucial for hormone regulation, inclusive of the balance of estrogen and other hormones.

Strategies:

ProbioticRich Foods: Such as yogurt, kefir, sauerkraut, and kimchi.

Prebiotic Foods: Include garlic, onions, bananas, and asparagus to feed useful intestine micro organism.

6. Stay Hydrated

Hydration and Hormones:

Proper hydration is critical for metabolic approaches and the stability of hormones.

FOODS THAT PROMOTE A HEALTHY GUT

Maintaining a wholesome gut is critical for typical properly being, as it affects digestion, immune feature, and even temper. A balanced and various gut microbiome can beautify nutrient absorption, guide weight control, and defend in opposition to numerous health issues.

1. Fermented Foods

Importance:

Fermented ingredients are wealthy in probiotics—beneficial micro organism that guide intestine fitness.

Examples:

Yogurt: Contains stay cultures like Lactobacillus and Bifidobacterium.

Kefir: A fermented dairy product with a various variety of probiotics.

Sauerkraut: Fermented cabbage that offers beneficial micro organism.

Kimchi: A spicy Korean aspect dish crafted from fermented veggies like cabbage and radishes.

Miso: A fermented soybean paste used in Japanese cuisine.

2. Prebiotic Foods

Importance:

Prebiotics are non digestible fibers that feed useful intestine micro organism, selling their boom and pastime.

Examples:

Garlic: Contains fructans that act as prebiotics.

Onions: Rich in insulin and fructooligosaccharides.

Bananas: Provide prebiotic fibers which include insulin and resistant starch.

Asparagus: Contains inulin and different prebiotic fibers.

Leeks: A excellent supply of prebiotic fibers like inulin.

3. High Fiber Foods

Importance:

Fiber supports digestion by using including bulk to stool and promoting ordinary bowel actions.

Examples:

Fruits: Apples, berries, and pears are excessive in soluble fiber.

Vegetables: Broccoli, carrots, and spinach offer diverse forms of fiber.

Whole Grains: Oats, quinoa, and brown rice are extremely good resources of dietary fiber.

Legumes: Beans, lentils, and chickpeas provide each soluble and insoluble fiber.

4. Omega3 Rich Foods

Importance:

Omegathree fatty acids have anti inflammatory residences that may gain intestine health and support the intestine lining.

Examples:

Fatty Fish: Salmon, mackerel, and sardines are high in omega3s.

Chia Seeds: A plant based supply of omega3s.

Flaxseeds: Rich in alphalinolenic acid (ALA), a sort of omega3 fatty acid.

Walnuts: Provide an amazing quantity of ALA.

5. Bone Broth

Importance:

Bone broth is rich in nutrients that assist intestine health, which includes collagen, gelatin, and amino acids.

Benefits:

Collagen and Gelatin: Help keep the integrity of the gut lining.

Amino Acids: Such as glycine and proline, support gut repair and characteristic.

6. Ginger

Importance:

Ginger has anti inflammatory and digestive blessings which can promote intestine health.

Benefits:

Soothes the Digestive Tract: Helps alleviate nausea and enhance digestion.

Reduces Inflammation: Can help overall gut fitness and luxury.

7. Turmeric

Importance:

Turmeric includes curcumin, a compound with anti inflammatory homes that could benefit intestine fitness.

Benefits:

Reduces Inflammation: Helps manage inflammation within the gut.

Supports Digestive Health: Promotes typical intestine comfort and function.

8. Leafy Greens

Importance:

Leafy veggies are high in vitamins, minerals, and fiber, assisting common intestine health.

Examples:

Spinach: Rich in fiber and nutrients like diet A and vitamin K.

Kale: Provides dietary fiber and antioxidants.

Swiss Chard: Contains fiber, nutrients, and minerals useful for gut fitness.

9. Herbs and Spices

Importance:

Certain herbs and spices have residences that may aid intestine health and digestion.

Examples:

Peppermint: Helps soothe digestive problems and alleviate bloating.

Cinnamon: Has antimicrobial residences that may gain gut health.

Fennel Seeds: Aid digestion and reduce bloating.

CHAPTER 2: THE SCIENCE OF EATING

MACRO NUTRIENTS AND MICRO NUTRIENTS

UNDERSTANDING PROTEINS, FATS, AND CARBOHYDRATES

Proteins, fats, and carbohydrates are the 3 macro nutrients that offer strength and are crucial for retaining various physical functions.

1. Proteins

Role in the Body:

Muscle Repair and Growth: Proteins are vital for building and repairing tissues, which includes muscular tissues.

Enzyme and Hormone Production: Proteins form enzymes that catalyze biochemical reactions and hormones that regulate diverse physiological tactics.

Immune Function: Proteins are involved in creating antibodies that assist combat infections.

Transport and Storage: Proteins help delivery vitamins and oxygen during the frame and shop crucial substances.

Sources:

Animal Based: Chicken, turkey, fish, red meat, eggs, and dairy products.

Plant Based: Beans, lentils, chickpeas, tofu, tempeh, and quinoa.

Types of Protein:

Complete Proteins: Contain all critical amino acids (e.G., animal products and quinoa).

Incomplete Proteins: Lack one or extra crucial amino acids (e.G., most plant primarily based proteins), but can be blended to shape complete proteins (e.G., beans and rice).

Daily Intake:

Recommended day by day allowance (RDA) is ready zero.8 grams according to kilogram of frame weight for the average adult. Needs may additionally vary primarily based on hobby stage, age, and health conditions.

2. Fats

Role within the Body:

Energy Storage: Fats provide a dense source of energy and are stored for future use.

Cell Structure: Fats are critical components of cellular membranes and contribute to their fluidity.

Hormone Production: Fats are involved in generating hormones, which include sex hormones and corticosteroids.

Insulation and Protection: Fat provides insulation and protects crucial organs from injury.

Types of Fat:

Saturated Fats: Found in animal products and some plant oils (e.G., coconut oil). Can raise LDL (bad) cholesterol levels if ate up in excess.

Unsaturated Fats: Found in plant oils, nuts, seeds, and fatty fish. Includes:

Monounsaturated Fats: Found in olive oil, avocados, and nuts. Can enhance heart health.

Polyunsaturated Fats: Found in fatty fish, flax seeds, and walnuts. Includes omega3 and omega6 fatty acids, which can be critical for heart fitness.

Trans Fats: Found in a few processed foods and margarine. Associated with accelerated danger of coronary heart disease and must be minimized.

Daily Intake:

Fats must make up about 2035% of your every day calorie intake. Emphasize unsaturated fat and restriction saturated and trans fats.

3. Carbohydrates

Role in the Body:

 Primary Energy Source: Carbohydrates are the frame's foremost source of strength, specially for the brain and muscle mass for the duration of exercise.

 Digestive Health: Fiber, a type of carbohydrate, supports digestive fitness and regular bowel moves.

 Regulation of Blood Sugar: Carbohydrates help regulate blood sugar levels via offering a consistent supply of electricity.

Types of Carbohydrates:

 Simple Carbohydrates: Consist of 1 or two sugar units and are quickly absorbed. Includes:

  Sugars: Found in end result, honey, and processed candies. Opt for natural sources like fruits.

 Complex Carbohydrates: Consist of a couple of sugar units and are digested extra slowly. Includes:

  Starches: Found in grains, legumes, and tubers (e.G., potatoes).

  Fiber: Found in end result, veggies, complete grains, and legumes. Benefits encompass advanced digestion and sustained energy degrees.

Daily Intake:

Carbohydrates ought to make up approximately 4565% of your each day calorie consumption. Focus on complicated carbohydrates and fiber wealthy ingredients for sustained energy and digestive health.

ESSENTIAL VITAMINS AND MINERALS FOR WEIGHT LOSS

While no unmarried diet or mineral will without delay lead to weight loss, certain vitamins play key roles in assisting metabolism, appetite law, and universal fitness, that can indirectly assist in weight control.

1. Vitamin D

Role in Weight Loss:

Metabolic Health: Helps regulate insulin and helps healthy blood sugar levels.

Fat Storage: May have an effect on fats garage and breakdown.

Sources:

Sunlight Exposure: The body can produce nutrition D while uncovered to daylight.

Foods: Fatty fish (e.G., salmon, mackerel), fortified dairy merchandise, egg yolks.

Supplementation:

Vitamin D3: Often endorsed for the ones who have restrained sun publicity or low tiers.

2. B Vitamins

Role in Weight Loss:

Energy Production: B vitamins, particularly B6, B12, and folate, are involved in converting food into strength.

Metabolism Regulation: Support wholesome metabolism and red blood cell formation.

Sources:

B6: Poultry, fish, bananas, potatoes.

B12: Meat, dairy products, eggs.

Folate: Leafy greens, legumes, fortified grains.

3. Vitamin C

Role in Weight Loss:

Antioxidant Protection: Helps defend cells from oxidative stress.

Metabolism Support: Plays a position in fat metabolism and the production of carnitine, that is critical for fat oxidation.

Sources:

Fruits: Oranges, strawberries, kiwi, and guava.

Vegetables: Bell peppers, broccoli, Brussels sprouts.

4. Calcium

Role in Weight Loss:

Fat Metabolism: May impact fat garage and the breakdown of fats cells.

Muscle Function: Supports muscle contraction and general metabolic function.

Sources:

Dairy Products: Milk, cheese, yogurt.

Plant Based Sources: Leafy greens (e.G., kale, collard vegetables), fortified plant milks, almonds.

5. Magnesium

Role in Weight Loss:

Energy Production: Involved in strength manufacturing and muscle function.

Blood Sugar Regulation: Helps adjust blood sugar tiers and might reduce insulin resistance.

Sources:

Nuts and Seeds: Almonds, pumpkin seeds.

Whole Grains: Brown rice, quinoa.

Leafy Greens: Spinach, Swiss chard.

6. Iron

Role in Weight Loss:

Oxygen Transport: Essential for the transport of oxygen within the blood, that is important for physical hobby and metabolism.

Energy Levels: Helps preserve strength stages and save you fatigue.

HOW TO MANAGE BLOOD SUGAR LEVELS FOR OPTIMAL WEIGHT LOSS

Maintaining strong blood sugar degrees is crucial for effective weight control and typical health. Fluctuating blood sugar levels can result in cravings, improved urge for food, and weight benefit.

1. Choose Low Glycemic Index (GI) Foods

Importance:

Low GI meals are digested more slowly, main to sluggish increases in blood sugar ranges and decreased insulin spikes.

Examples of Low GI Foods:

Whole Grains: Quinoa, barley, and metal reduce oats.

Non Starchy Vegetables: Spinach, broccoli, and cauliflower.

Legumes: Beans, lentils, and chickpeas.

Fruits: Berries, apples, and pears.

2. Incorporate FiberRich Foods

Importance:

Fiber facilitates gradual down the digestion and absorption of carbohydrates, main to greater strong blood sugar stages.

Sources of Fiber:

Vegetables: Leafy veggies, carrots, and bell peppers.

Fruits: Apples, oranges, and strawberries.

Whole Grains: Oats, brown rice, and entire wheat bread.

Legumes: Lentils, black beans, and chickpeas.

3. Combine Carbohydrates with Protein and Healthy Fats

Importance:

Combining carbohydrates with protein and fat can gradual down the absorption of glucose, supporting to keep stable blood sugar stages.

Examples:

Snack Ideas: Apple slices with almond butter or yogurt with berries and nuts.

Meal Ideas: Quinoa salad with greens, grilled chicken, and avocado.

4. Eat Regular, Balanced Meals

Importance:

Regular food prevent extreme fluctuations in blood sugar ranges and assist control starvation and cravings.

HOW CALORIC DENSITY AFFECTS HUNGER AND FULLNESS

Caloric density, also called strength density, refers back to the range of energy in a given weight or volume of food. Foods with extraordinary caloric densities have an effect on hunger and fullness in numerous approaches.

1. Low Caloric Density Foods

Characteristics:

High in Water and Fiber: Foods which includes fruits, greens, and soups are frequently low in energy but excessive in water and fiber.

Bulk and Volume: These foods provide larger portions for fewer energy, which could help fill the stomach.

Effects on Hunger and Fullness:

Increased Satiety: Low caloric density ingredients can sell a sense of fullness because they absorb greater space in the belly.

Reduced Caloric Intake: Eating those meals can help manipulate normal calorie intake without feeling disadvantaged or hungry.

Examples:

Vegetables: Leafy greens, cucumbers, and tomatoes.

Fruits: Apples, berries, and oranges.

Soups: Broth based totally soups with plenty of veggies.

2. High Caloric Density Foods

Characteristics:

High in Fat and Sugar: Foods which include nuts, oils, and pastries are excessive in calories but low in volume.

Compact and Dense: These ingredients provide a small quantity of food for a huge quantity of energy.

Effects on Hunger and Fullness:

Less Satiety: High caloric density ingredients won't fill the stomach as effectively, main to quicker returns of starvation.

Higher Caloric Intake: Consuming these foods can result in accelerated calorie consumption with out feeling full, which can contribute to weight gain if now not controlled properly.

Examples:

Nuts and Seeds: Almonds, peanuts, and sunflower seeds.

Oils and Butters: Olive oil, butter, and margarine.

Pastries and Snack Foods: Cookies, chips, and sweet.

3. Strategies for Managing Hunger and Fullness

Incorporate More Low Caloric Density Foods:

Focus on Vegetables: Fill 1/2 of your plate with vegetables, which can be low in energy however excessive in vitamins and fiber.

Eat More Fruits: Choose culmination as snacks or desserts to meet candy cravings even as staying within calorie limits.

Balance High Caloric Density Foods:

Moderation: Include high caloric density meals in small portions to keep away from immoderate calorie consumption.

Bankruptcy : Building Your Diet Plan

CHAPTER 3: SETTING REALISTIC GOALS

ESTABLISHING ATTAINABLE WEIGHT LOSS AND HEALTH GOALS

Setting sensible and viable weight loss and health goals is crucial for lengthy term success. Goals must be precise, measurable, conceivable, relevant, and time sure (SMART).

1. Define Your Goals Clearly

Weight Loss Goals:

Specific: Clearly kingdom how a lot weight you want to lose (e.G., 10 pounds).

Measurable: Set milestones to music progress (e.G., lose 12 kilos in line with week).

Health Goals:

Specific: Define what you want to gain (e.G., lower blood stress, boom fitness level).

Measurable: Use metrics like blood pressure readings, fitness checks, or dietary changes.

2. Ensure Goals Are Attainable

Realistic Expectations:

Rate of Weight Loss: Aim for 12 kilos in line with week, which is a wholesome and sustainable rate.

Lifestyle Changes: Set desires that in shape inside your current way of life and assets (e.G., incorporating a 30minute stroll daily).

Consider Barriers:

Time Constraints: Set goals that fit together with your agenda and commitments.

Resource Availability: Ensure you've got get entry to to the necessary resources (e.G., healthful ingredients, health club get entry to).

3. Make Goals Relevant

Align with Your Values:

Personal Motivation: Choose dreams that resonate together with your nonpublic values and motivations (e.G., enhancing strength degrees, enhancing overall nicely being).

Long Term Benefits: Focus on health improvements that contribute in your longtime period high quality of life.

Avoid Unrealistic Comparisons:

Individual Differences: Set dreams based totally on your personal needs and circumstances in place of evaluating to others.

4. Set a Timeline

Short Term Goals:

Immediate Steps: Set goals for the next 13 months (e.G., losing 5 kilos, drinking extra water every day).

Long Term Goals:

Extended Vision: Set dreams for 6three hundred and sixty five days or longer (e.G., accomplishing a goal weight, strolling a 5K).

Review and Adjust:

Regular Checkins: Assess your progress periodically and adjust your dreams as wished based in your achievements and demanding situations.

5. Develop an Action Plan

Dietary Changes:

Healthy Eating: Incorporate balanced food with lean proteins, complete grains, end result, and vegetables.

Portion Control: Practice aware consuming and portion manipulate to manage calorie consumption.

HOW TO CREATE BALANCED, NUTRITIOUS MEALS

Creating balanced, nutritious meals entails incorporating a whole lot of meals groups to ensure you get vital nutrients, assist typical health, and preserve electricity degrees.

1. Understand the Components of a Balanced Meal

1.1. Protein

Role: Builds and upkeep tissues, supports immune function, and continues you complete.

Sources: Lean meats (hen, turkey), fish, eggs, dairy products, legumes (beans, lentils), tofu, and tempeh.

1.2. Carbohydrates

Role: Provides energy and helps mind function.

Sources: Whole grains (brown rice, quinoa, oats), fruits, veggies, and legumes. Opt for complicated carbohydrates over refined ones for sustained energy.

1.3. Fats

Role: Supports mobile shape, hormone production, and nutrient absorption.

Sources: Healthy fat from avocados, nuts, seeds, olive oil, and fatty fish (salmon, mackerel).

1.4. Vegetables

Role: Provides nutrients, minerals, fiber, and antioxidants.

Sources: A sort of colorful vegetables like spinach, broccoli, bell peppers, and carrots.

1.Five. Fruits

Role: Offers vitamins, minerals, fiber, and natural sweetness.

Sources: Fresh culmination like apples, berries, oranges, and bananas.

1.6. Fluids

Role: Supports hydration, digestion, and universal physical functions.

Sources: Water, natural teas, and broth based soups.

2. Plan Your Meals

2.1. Portion Control

Protein: Aim for a serving size of 3four ounces of lean protein.

Carbohydrates: Half of your plate must be full of complex carbohydrates.

Vegetables: Aim for at least half of of your plate to be veggies.

Fats: Use fat carefully, aiming for about 12 tablespoons of healthful fat in step with meal.

READING AND UNDERSTANDING FOOD
LABELS

Food labels offer critical records approximately the nutritional content material of packaged ingredients. Understanding a way to examine those labels permit you to make healthier picks and higher control your eating regimen.

1. Serving Size

What to Look For:

Serving Size: The quantity of food or drink that is considered one serving. This is typically listed in each general measurements (e.G., cups, oz) and in grams.

Servings Per Container: Indicates what number of servings are within the entire package.

Why It Matters:

Portion Control: Helps you recognize what number of calories and nutrients you devour in keeping with serving. Be aware that consuming more than one serving will increase your intake of energy, fat, sugars, and many others.

2. Calories

What to Look For:

Calories in line with Serving: Shows the full quantity of energy you'll devour in a single serving of the product.

Why It Matters:

Energy Balance: Helps you manipulate your every day calorie consumption. For weight control, it's essential to stability energy ate up with calories burned.

3. Nutritional Content

3.1. Nutrients to Limit

Total Fat: Includes saturated fat and trans fat. High intake of those fats can boom the danger of coronary heart disease.

Cholesterol: High levels can affect heart health.

Sodium: Excess sodium can contribute to excessive blood pressure.

3.2. Nutrients to Get Enough Of

Dietary Fiber: Promotes digestive fitness and might resource in weight control.

Protein: Essential for muscle restore and ordinary health.

Vitamins and Minerals: Look for key nutrients including nutrition A, nutrition C, calcium, and iron.

CHAPTER 4: EATING STRATEGIES

MINDFUL EATING

THE BENEFITS OF MINDFUL EATING PRACTICES

Mindful eating includes paying complete attention to the eating revel in, focusing at the flavors, textures, and sensations of meals, and being aware about your body's hunger and fullness cues.

1. Improved Digestion

How It Helps:

Slows Down Eating: Eating slowly and chewing thoroughly can aid digestion through giving your digestive machine greater time to procedure food.

Increases Satiety: Mindful ingesting facilitates you understand while you're complete, which can prevent overeating and decrease the danger of digestive soreness.

Benefits:

Better Nutrient Absorption: Proper chewing and slower consuming can beautify the breakdown of food, making vitamins extra on hand for your frame.

2. Weight Management

How It Helps:

Reduces Overeating: By being greater privy to hunger and fullness cues, you are much less possibly to consume past your physical desires.

Promotes Portion Control: Mindful ingesting encourages you to pay attention for your frame's indicators in place of ingesting out of dependency or emotion.

Benefits:

Sustainable Weight Loss: Helps in accomplishing and keeping a wholesome weight through fostering a healthier relationship with meals.

INTERMITTENT FASTING

Intermittent Fasting: An Overview

Intermittent fasting (IF) is an eating sample that alternates among intervals of fasting and eating. It makes a speciality of while you devour as opposed to what you consume. Here's a complete guide to knowledge intermittent fasting, consisting of its advantages, methods, and issues.

1. What is Intermittent Fasting?

Intermittent fasting includes biking between periods of fasting and eating. It does no longer prescribe specific foods but emphasizes the timing of your food. Common techniques consist of:

1.1. sixteen/eight Method

Structure: Fast for 16 hours and devour all through an 8hour window (e.G., eat from 12 PM to eight PM).

Popularity: One of the maximum broadly practiced intermittent fasting methods.

1.2. 5:2 Diet

Structure: Eat typically for five days of the week and restriction calorie consumption to approximately 500six hundred energy on the opposite 2 nonconsecutive days.

Flexibility: Allows for normal consuming on most days with periodic calorie reduction.

1.3. Eat Stop Eat

Structure: Fast for twenty four hours a couple of times every week (e.G., from dinner one day to dinner the next day).

Intensity: More challenging because of the prolonged fasting duration.

1.4. Alternate Day Fasting

Structure: Alternate between days of ordinary consuming and days of fasting or very low calorie consumption.

Variety: Offers flexibility in fasting frequency.

1.5. Warrior Diet

Structure: Fast for 20 hours and devour one huge meal in a fourhour window.

Focus: Emphasizes eating in the nighttime and eating small quantities of uncooked fruits and vegetables during the fasting period.

2. Benefits of Intermittent Fasting

2.1. Weight Loss and Fat Loss

Caloric Intake: Restricts eating windows, that may result in decreased calorie consumption and weight reduction.

Metabolic Rate: May boom metabolism through hormone law, consisting of accelerated norepinephrine degrees.

2.2. Improved Insulin Sensitivity

Blood Sugar Regulation: Helps decrease blood sugar tiers and improve insulin sensitivity, probably reducing the hazard of kind 2 diabetes.

2.3. Enhanced Cellular Repair

: Eating Out and Social Situations

Eating Out and Social Situations: Tips for MAINTAINING A HEALTHY DIET

Eating out and navigating social conditions can gift demanding situations whilst seeking to hold a healthful diet. However, with a bit of making plans and mindfulness, you could make picks that align with your dietary desires while nonetheless playing social interactions.

1. Planning Ahead

1.1. Research Restaurant Menus

Pre Check Options: Many eating places offer their menus online. Review alternatives beforehand to pick out healthier selections or to devise the way to make changes.

Look for Nutritional Information: Some restaurants provide dietary information for their dishes, which allow you to make knowledgeable alternatives.

1.2. Make a Strategy

Set Goals: Determine what you want to obtain (e.G., sticking to a calorie restriction, choosing low carb alternatives) and plan your alternatives consequently.

Decide on Portions: Decide in case you'll order an appetizer and principal route or just one dish, and whether you'll choose smaller portions or percentage dishes.

2. Choosing Healthy Options

2.1. Prioritize Nutrient Dense Foods

Lean Proteins: Opt for grilled, baked, or steamed proteins which includes chook, fish, or tofu.

Vegetables: Choose dishes with a lot of vegetables or order a facet salad along with your meal.

2.2. Watch Portions

Portion Control: Consider ordering a smaller portion or sharing dishes to manipulate portion sizes.

Be Mindful of Extras: Avoid excessive calorie extras like creamy sauces, fried objects, or excessive cheese.

2.3. Modify Your Order

Ask for Changes: Request adjustments along with dressing on the facet, grilling rather than frying, or substituting healthier sides.

Request Ingredients: Ask approximately how dishes are organized or what ingredients are used to keep away from hidden calories or dangerous fat.

3. Managing Social Situations

3.1. Practice Mindful Eating

 Slow Down: Eat slowly and relish each chew, which facilitates you apprehend starvation and fullness cues.

 Listen to Your Body: Pay interest to how complete you experience and stop ingesting whilst you're glad, not just when your plate is empty.

CHAPTER 5: LIFESTYLE INTEGRATION

EXERCISE AND PHYSICAL ACTIVITY

THE ROLE OF EXERCISE IN WEIGHT LOSS AND HEALTH

Exercise performs a essential role in accomplishing and keeping weight reduction, as well as supporting overall fitness and well being.

1. Weight Loss and Management

1.1. Calorie Expenditure

Burning Calories: Exercise increases the number of energy you burn, which can help create a calorie deficit vital for weight loss.

Types of Exercise: Both aerobic (aerobic) sports (e.G., going for walks, cycling) and strength training (e.G., weight lifting) make a contribution to calorie burning.

1.2. Metabolic Rate

Boosts Metabolism: Regular bodily pastime can boom your resting metabolic price, helping you burn greater calories at relaxation.

Muscle Mass: Strength education builds muscle, which can beautify metabolic price when you consider that muscle groups burns more calories than fats tissue.

1.3. Fat Loss vs. Muscle Gain

Body Composition: Exercise facilitates to reduce body fat even as maintaining or growing muscles, main to a more fit frame composition.

Fat Distribution: Helps in reducing visceral fat (fats round inner organs) which is linked to diverse fitness risks.

2. Health Benefits Beyond Weight Loss

2.1. Cardiovascular Health

Heart Health: Regular exercising strengthens the coronary heart, improves movement, and helps lower blood strain and cholesterol levels.

Reduced Risk of Disease: Regular physical interest can reduce the risk of heart disorder, stroke, and type 2 diabetes.

2.2. Mental Health

Mood Enhancement: Exercise releases endorphins, that may enhance mood and reduce emotions of tension and despair.

Stress Reduction: Physical interest enables manipulate pressure and improves universal mental well being.

2.Three. Bone and Muscle Health

Bone Density: Weight bearing exercises (e.G., strolling, jogging) support bones and can help save you osteoporosis.

Muscle Strength: Building muscle via electricity education improves useful electricity and reduces the risk of injury.

STRESS MANAGEMENT AND SLEEP

Creating an Exercise Routine That Works for You Developing an workout habitual that suits your way of life and goals is essential for long term achievement.

1. Assess Your Fitness Level and Goals

1.1. Evaluate Your Current Fitness Level

Fitness Assessment: Determine your current level of fitness by means of assessing strength, staying power, flexibility, and cardiovascular fitness.

Identify Limitations: Consider any bodily limitations or fitness troubles which could have an effect on your workout picks.

1.2. Set Clear, Achievable Goals

Short Term Goals: Focus on immediately objectives which includes improving patience, power, or flexibility.

Long Term Goals: Set broader dreams like losing weight, building muscle, or enhancing standard health.

2. Choose Activities You Enjoy

2.1. Identify Preferred Exercises

Personal Preferences: Select physical games you locate enjoyable, whether or not it's jogging, swimming, dancing, or trekking.

Experiment: Try one of a kind sports to find out what you experience most.

2.2. Incorporate Variety

Mix It Up: Include a combination of aerobic, electricity, flexibility, and stability sports to prevent boredom and work special muscle companies.

Seasonal Activities: Adapt your habitual to encompass seasonal activities or sports activities.

3. Design a Balanced Routine

3.1. Plan Workout Frequency

Consistency: Aim for at the least 150 minutes of slight depth or seventy five minutes of excessive depth aerobic exercising consistent with week, mixed with muscle strengthening sports on two or extra days.

Frequency: Decide what number of days per week you may realistically decide to exercise.

3.2. Determine Workout Duration

Session Length: Plan for exercise periods that healthy into your agenda, whether they're 30 minutes or an hour.

Flexibility: Incorporate shorter, excessive intensity exercises if time is confined.

3.3. Balance Different Types of Exercise

Cardiovascular: Include activities like strolling, biking, or swimming to improve heart health and persistence.

Strength Training: Add exercises like weight lifting, resistance bands, or body weight sports to build muscle and energy.

Flexibility and Balance: Incorporate stretching, yoga, or Pilates to improve flexibility and stability.

4. Create a Workout Schedule

four.1. Set a Routine

Consistency: Schedule your workouts on the equal time every day to construct a ordinary.

Flexibility: Adjust your time table as had to accommodate changes in your lifestyle or commitments.

4.2. Include Rest and Recovery

Rest Days: Incorporate relaxation days or lighter hobby days to allow your body to recover and prevent over training.

Active Recovery: Consider low intensity activities like walking or gentle stretching on rest days.

5. Track Progress and Adjust

5.1. Monitor Your Progress

Track Workouts: Use a health app or magazine to log your exercises, song progress, and live encouraged.

Measure Success: Track enhancements in strength, persistence, flexibility, or frame composition.

5.2. Adjust as Needed

Adapt Routine: Modify your habitual based on development, changing goals, or comments from your frame.

Set New Goals: Regularly reexamine your goals and set new challenges to keep your ordinary enticing.

6. Stay Motivated and Engaged

6.1. Find a Workout Buddy

Support System: Exercise with a chum or be a part of a health institution to stay prompted and accountable.

Social Aspect: Enjoy the social benefits of working out with others.

6.2. Incorporate Rewards

Celebrate Achievements: Reward yourself for reaching milestones or sticking on your routine.

Enjoyable Activities: Include sports you like or deal with your self to something unique as a reward.

Stress Management and Sleep

How strain and sleep affect weight reduction

Stress and sleep play large roles in weight control and general health. Understanding how they impact weight reduction allow you to address these factors to gain higher consequences.

1. The Impact of Stress on Weight Loss

1.1. Hormonal Changes

Cortisol: Chronic pressure ends in improved cortisol ranges, a hormone related to accelerated appetite and cravings for excessive calorie, sugary ingredients. This can make a contribution to weight advantage, especially around the stomach place.

Insulin Resistance: Stress can result in insulin resistance, affecting your frame's capacity to alter blood sugar tiers, that can impact weight control.

1.2. Emotional Eating

Comfort Eating: Stress often triggers emotional consuming, where individuals flip to meals for comfort in preference to starvation. This can lead to eating extra calories and dangerous foods.

Cravings: High pressure can growth cravings for comfort foods high in sugar and fat, main to over consumption and weight benefit.

1.3. Metabolic Effects

Altered Metabolism: Stress can disrupt normal metabolic methods, probably leading to accelerated fat garage and reduced muscular tissues, which influences weight loss efforts.

Reduced Physical Activity: Stress may additionally cause fatigue or loss of motivation, reducing bodily activity tiers and hindering weight loss.

1.4. Sleep Disruption

 Quality of Sleep: Stress often influences sleep best and length, developing a cycle that in addition exacerbates weight management issues.

 2. The Impact of Sleep on Weight Loss

2.1. Hormonal Regulation

 Leptin and Ghrelin: Sleep deprivation can disrupt the balance of hunger regulating hormones leptin and ghrelin. Leptin, which indicators satiety, decreases, while ghrelin, which stimulates urge for food, increases, main to accelerated hunger and calorie intake.

 Insulin Sensitivity: Poor sleep can impair insulin sensitivity, making it more difficult to your body to manage blood sugar degrees and increasing the threat of weight benefit.

2.2. Metabolism

 Resting Metabolic Rate: Inadequate sleep can decrease your resting metabolic price (RMR), which means you burn fewer calories at relaxation. This can gradual down weight reduction and make a contribution to weight benefit.

Fat Storage: Sleep deprivation has been linked to increased fats garage and reduced fat oxidation, making it greater challenging to shed pounds.

2.3. Appetite Control

Increased Appetite: Lack of sleep frequently results in accelerated urge for food and cravings for high calorie ingredients, contributing to weight advantage.

Food Choices: Sleep deprived individuals may also make poorer food selections, opting for dangerous snacks and large portions.

2.4. Physical Activity

Energy Levels: Poor sleep can cause reduced energy tiers and motivation, decreasing the likelihood of undertaking everyday bodily pastime.

Exercise Performance: Lack of sleep can negatively effect workout overall performance, making workouts much less effective and doubtlessly hindering weight reduction.

3. Strategies for Managing Stress and Improving Sleep

3.1. Stress Management Techniques

Mindfulness and Relaxation: Practice mindfulness, meditation, or deep respiratory physical activities to lessen stress tiers.

Exercise: Regular bodily hobby can assist manipulate stress and improve mood.

Healthy Coping Strategies: Develop wholesome methods to deal with stress, such as conducting pastimes, spending time with loved ones, or searching for guide from a counselor.